MACULAR DEGENERATION DIET COOKBOOK

Delicious, Nutrient-Rich Recipes To Support Eye Health, Improve Vision, Boost Immune System And More – All You Need To Know

DR. AMARI VALERIE

TABLE OF CONTENTS

BONUS:

7 days meal plan recipes, ingredients, and detailed preparatory guidelines for Macular Degeneration

7 Desserts procedural recipes for Macular Degeneration and guidelines

7 Smoothies procedural recipes for Macular Degeneration and guidelines

DISCLAIMER

The information provided in this book, is for educational and informational purposes only and is not intended as medical advice. The content is not a substitute for professional medical advice, diagnosis, or treatment. Always seek the advice of your physician or other qualified health provider with any questions you may have regarding a medical condition. Never disregard professional medical advice or delay in seeking it because of something you have read in this book.

The dietary suggestions and recipes in this book are based on general guidelines and may not be suitable for everyone. Individual responses to foods can vary, and it is important to consult with a healthcare professional before making any significant changes to your diet.

The author and publisher of this book do not claim to cure or treat any medical condition. The information provided is based on research and personal experience and is intended to help readers make informed decisions about their diet and health.

Furthermore, I the author do not endorse any specific products, brands, treatments, or services that may be mentioned in this book. Any references to products, services, websites, or organizations are provided for informational purposes only and do not constitute an endorsement or recommendation by the author. The inclusion of such references does not imply any association, sponsorship, or affiliation between the author and the referenced entities.

The recipes and dietary suggestions in this book are designed to be safe and healthful. However, readers should use their own discretion and consult with a healthcare professional when necessary, especially if they have allergies, sensitivities, or other dietary restrictions.

By using this book, you acknowledge and agree that the author and publisher shall not be held liable for any loss or damage, including but not limited to special, incidental, consequential, or other damages, resulting from the use of the information and recipes contained in this book.

ABOUT THIS BOOK

This "Macular Degeneration Diet Cookbook" is an exhaustive guide that is intended to provide support to individuals who are coping with macular degeneration by facilitating dietary adjustments. This book is essential for individuals who wish to effectively manage their condition while simultaneously consuming nutritious, delectable meals. It commences with a perceptive overview of macular degeneration, which encompasses its definition, categories, symptoms, and risk factors.

The significance of early detection and management is underscored, as this condition can have a significant impact on daily life and vision. This book emphasizes the substantial impact that diet can have on eye health, thereby allowing for a more in-depth examination of the role of nutrition in the management of macular degeneration.

The significance of nutrition in eye health is meticulously delineated, highlighting the critical nutrients, such as antioxidants, vitamins, and minerals, that are essential for the preservation of vision. This book delineates the direct impact of diet on the progression of macular degeneration, underscoring the importance of hydration and the advantages of particular nutrients on overall health. Readers will acquire a comprehensive comprehension of how to incorporate these indispensable components into their daily diets, thereby guaranteeing that their diets effectively promote their eye health.

The following are practical guidelines for a diet that is conducive to macular degeneration. These guidelines include a list of foods to include and exclude, meal preparation advice, and strategies for interpreting food labels and nutritional information. This book underscores the significance of balance and diversity, providing strategies for integrating a diverse array of nutrients into one's diet. It also offers guidance on the safe and efficient preparation of meals, the preservation of nutrient content, and the use of wise grocery purchasing strategies, thereby empowering readers to make well-informed dietary decisions.

This book addresses frequently inquired questions and common concerns, including the necessity of supplements and the possibility of curing macular degeneration through diet alone. It provides advice on how to manage dietary changes in conjunction with other health conditions and how to address dietary restrictions and allergies.

This comprehensive approach guarantees that readers experience a sense of support and information as they progress through their dietary voyage.

The chapters that are devoted to recipes offer a plethora of choices for each meal, ranging from nutrient-rich breakfasts to satisfying dinners. Each recipe is intended to be both palatable and advantageous to ocular health, utilizing ingredients that are abundant in essential nutrients. This book provides readers with the necessary tools to easily implement the dietary adjustments suggested, such as procedural guidelines, specific recipes for snacking, desserts, and smoothies, and detailed meal plans.

In essence, this "Macular Degradation Diet Cookbook" is an invaluable resource for individuals who are interested in managing macular degeneration through diet. It empowers readers to be in control of their ocular health sustainably and enjoyably by integrating practical advice, delectable recipes, and scientific insights.

CHAPTER ONE

Introduction

The introduction establishes the foundation for the subsequent chapters, introducing readers to the realm of macular degeneration and the role of diet in its management. It prepares readers for the forthcoming content by underscoring the significance of dietary choices in promoting eye health and overall well-being.

Comprehending Macular Degeneration

In this section, readers explore the specifics of macular degeneration, acquiring an exhaustive understanding of its implications. This section establishes a firm foundation for understanding the intricacies of macular degeneration, encompassing the morphology of the eye and the underlying mechanisms.

Dietary Interventions For Macular Degeneration

Readers are provided with practical advice on how to incorporate dietary modifications to promote eye health in this section. Readers are provided with actionable steps to maximize their diet for macular degeneration management, including the incorporation of nutrient-rich foods such as leafy greens, colorful fruits, and omega-3 fatty acids, as well as the reduction of processed foods and saturated fats.

Meal Plans And Recipes

This section provides a diverse selection of delectable recipes and meal plans that are specifically designed for individuals with macular degeneration, with an emphasis on simplicity and accessibility. These recipes emphasize both nutrition and flavor to create a joyful experience of healthy eating, from vibrant salads that are brimming with antioxidants to hearty soups that are rich in vitamins and minerals.

Lifestyle Advice And Resources

This section completes the cookbook by offering valuable lifestyle advice and supplementary resources to assist individuals in their pursuit of improved eye health. This section provides readers with the resources necessary to thrive in the face of macular degeneration, including practical advice on meal preparation and grocery purchasing, as well as recommendations for additional reading and community support groups.

Role Of Nutrition In Eye Health

Nutrition is essential for the preservation of healthy eyes, particularly in the context of macular degeneration. Essential vitamins and minerals that are essential for eye health can be obtained by incorporating nutrient-rich foods into one's diet. Foods that are abundant in antioxidants, omega-3 fatty acids, and vitamins A, C, and E can assist in safeguarding the eyes from the effects of free radicals and aging. By emphasizing a well-rounded diet that encompasses a diverse array of fruits, vegetables, whole cereals, lean proteins, and healthy lipids, it is possible to enhance overall eye health and mitigate the risk of macular degeneration progression.

Essential Nutrients For Eye Health

Several nutrients are crucial for the preservation of optimal eye health, particularly in the prevention or halting of macular degeneration. Leafy greens, such as spinach and kale, contain lutein and zeaxanthin, which provide retinal protection from oxidative stress and hazardous blue light. Omega-3 fatty acids, which are present in fatty fish such as mackerel and salmon, are known to promote retinal function and alleviate inflammation. Vitamin C, which is abundant in citrus fruits and berries, enhances collagen production and fortifies blood vessels in the conjunctiva. Furthermore, vitamin E, which is present in nuts and seeds, functions as a potent antioxidant, safeguarding cells from harm.

The Impact Of Diet On Macular Degeneration

The development and progression of macular degeneration are significantly influenced by diet. Damage to the macula can result from the consumption of processed foods, refined carbohydrates, and unhealthy lipids, which can contribute to inflammation and oxidative stress in the body.

In contrast, a diet that is abundant in whole, nutrient-dense foods can assist in the reduction of inflammation, the prevention of oxidative damage, and the promotion of overall eye health. Individuals can potentially delay the progression of macular degeneration and reduce their risk of developing it by making mindful choices and prioritizing nutrient-rich foods.

The Advantages Of Antioxidants

Antioxidants are essential for the preservation of ocular health and are essential in the prevention of macular degeneration. These compounds are capable of neutralizing free radicals, which are unstable molecules that can inflict harm on the cells and tissues of the eye.

Berries, citrus, carrots, and bell peppers are among the colorful fruits and vegetables that are high in antioxidants. The risk of macular degeneration can be mitigated by consuming a diet that is rich in antioxidants, which safeguard the retina from oxidative stress and inflammation. Furthermore, antioxidants may have anti-aging effects on the eyes and promote overall health.

Vitamins And Minerals Are Essential For Vision

Maintaining optimal vision and safeguarding against macular degeneration necessitates the consumption of numerous vitamins and minerals. Vitamin A, which is present in orange and yellow fruits and vegetables, is crucial for the preservation of a healthy retina and the ability to see in the dark.

Citrus fruits and verdant greens are rich in vitamin C, which is essential for the health of blood vessels in the eyes and the prevention of age-related eye diseases. Vitamin E is a potent antioxidant that safeguards cells from harm and is present in almonds, seeds, and vegetable oils.

In addition, the consumption of minerals such as zinc and copper as part of a well-balanced diet can mitigate the progression of macular degeneration and contribute to retinal function.

CHAPTER TWO

Macular Degeneration-Friendly Dietary Recommendations

Focus on the inclusion of foods that are high in antioxidants, vitamins A, C, and E, zinc, lutein, zeaxanthin, and omega-3 fatty acids when developing a diet that is appropriate for macular degeneration.

Encourage the consumption of colorful fruits and vegetables, including carrots, spinach, kale, and berries, as well as fish that are rich in omega-3s, such as mackerel and salmon. Choose lean proteins, whole cereals, and healthful fats, such as those found in nuts and seeds.

Foods to Incorporate into Your Diet: To guarantee a diverse intake of essential nutrients, consume a variety of colorful fruits and vegetables.

For instance, enjoy a colorful salad with mixed berries, incorporate spinach into your morning omelet, or graze on vegetables with hummus. Support eye health by incorporating sources of omega-3 fatty acids, including sardines, walnuts, flaxseeds, and salmon. For sustained energy and fiber, opt for whole grains such as brown rice, quinoa, and whole wheat bread.

Foods to Avoid: Consume limited quantities of foods that are high in saturated and trans fats, as they can contribute to oxidative stress and inflammation in the body. Refrain from consuming an excessive amount of red meat, saccharine treats, or processed and fried foods.

Reduce the consumption of refined carbohydrates, such as white bread, pasta, and confectionary, as they have the potential to elevate blood sugar levels and induce inflammation.

Furthermore, it is recommended that sodium ingestion be reduced to preserve optimal blood pressure levels.

Meal Planning and Preparation Advice: To guarantee that you have a variety of nutritious alternatives at your disposal, plan your meals. To simplify meal preparation throughout the week, batch cook cereals, proteins, and vegetables. To preserve nutrients without the addition of excessive lipids, experiment with various culinary methods, such as grilling, roasting, and steaming. Incorporate herbs and seasonings to improve the flavor of a dish without the use of salt. Incorporate a diverse array of colors, textures, and flavors to develop well-rounded meals.

Understanding Nutritional Information and Food Labels: To identify nutrient-dense, whole foods, concentrate on the ingredients list when reading food labels. Search for products that contain minimal amounts of artificial additives, unhealthy lipids, and added sugars.

To prevent the overconsumption of calories and nutrients, it is important to be mindful of serving sizes. Compare various brands to select those that are higher in fiber and lower in sodium. Make informed decisions that promote eye wellness and overall health by utilizing nutritional information.

Cooking Tips And Kitchen Essentials

It is imperative to have the appropriate kitchen utensils when beginning a macular degeneration diet to prepare nutritious meals. Invest in a high-quality blender to create smoothies that are rich in antioxidants, which are beneficial for eye health. Another valuable instrument for cooking vegetables while preserving their nutrients is a sterilizer. Furthermore, it is advisable to acquire a mandoline slicer to effortlessly slice fruits and vegetables into thin, precise pieces, which are ideal for salads and snacking. To guarantee the safety and efficiency of meal preparation, it is crucial to maintain a clean and organized kitchen and to adhere to appropriate food handling practices to prevent contamination.

To promote ocular health, it is recommended to use cooking oils that are high in omega-3 fatty acids, such as olive oil. Lastly, when restocking your larder and refrigerator, prioritize whole cereals, lean proteins, and an abundance of vibrant fruits and vegetables.

When purchasing supplies for your macular degeneration diet, prioritize the inclusion of nutrient-dense foods that promote eye health in your cart. Begin by accumulating verdant greens such as spinach, kale, and collard greens, which are abundant in antioxidants such as zeaxanthin and lutein.

Opt for vibrant fruits, including kiwi, oranges, and berries, which are rich in vitamins C and E, which are crucial for the preservation of healthy vision. It is important to incorporate omega-3-rich foods, such as mackerel, walnuts, and salmon, into your diet to mitigate the risk of macular degeneration progression.

Choose whole cereals such as quinoa, brown rice, and oats to obtain essential nutrients and fiber. Lastly, it is important to carefully read food labels to avoid products that are high in sodium, added sugars, and saturated fats, as these can have a detrimental effect on ocular health.

Essential Kitchen Equipment For Healthier Cooking

Providing your kitchen with the necessary instruments can simplify and enhance the experience of healthful cooking for macular degeneration. Invest in a high-speed blender, which is ideal for creating nutrient-rich smoothies with ingredients such as berries, almonds, and leafy vegetables.

A cutting board supplies a stable surface for food preparation, while a high-quality chef's knife is essential for precise slicing of vegetables and fruits. When cooking vegetables, it is advisable to invest in a steamer container to maintain their nutrients and texture. A non-stick skillet is an excellent choice for preparing fish, poultry, and eggs with minimal additional fat. Finally, ensure that you have measuring glasses and utensils on hand to ensure that you can accurately measure ingredients and control your portions when following recipes.

Hints For The Safe And Efficient Preparation Of Meals

Efficient meal preparation is essential for adhering to a macular degeneration diet. Begin by scheduling your meals and refreshments for the upcoming week, ensuring that you include nutrient-dense foods such as leafy greens, vibrant fruits, and omega-3-rich proteins.

During the hectic weekdays, it is possible to save time by prepping ingredients in advance, such as rinsing and slicing vegetables. To preserve the nutrients in foods without introducing additional oil, employ culinary methods such as steaming, baking, and grilling. To maintain the freshness of leftovers and minimize food waste, store them in hermetic containers in the refrigerator. Additionally, it is imperative to adhere to safe food handling practices, including the use of separate cutting boards for uncooked meat and produce to prevent cross-contamination and the cleansing of hands before and after handling food.

Methods For Preserving The Nutrient Content Of Foods

It is essential to maintain the nutrient content of foods to optimize the advantages of a macular degeneration diet. Choose cooking methods such as steaming, sautéing, and microwaving, which are more nutrient-dense than simmering or frying. To help preserve the vitamins and minerals in vegetables, strive for a crisp-tender texture during the preparation process. Foods should not be overcooked, as protracted exposure to heat can lead to the degradation of nutrients. To optimize the nutritional value of vegetables, it is recommended that they be incorporated into salads or treats that are minimally cooked or fresh.

Furthermore, it is crucial to store fruits and vegetables in a manner that preserves their nutritional value and freshness. To prevent spoilage, store root vegetables such as potatoes and onions in a cold, dark place and keep perishable items like fruit and leafy greens in the refrigerator.

CHAPTER THREE

Frequently Asked Questions And Common Concerns

Many individuals are uncertain as to whether macular degeneration can be cured solely through diet. Although a nutritious diet can undoubtedly promote eye health and potentially impede the progression of the disease, it is improbable that it will completely eradicate it. Nevertheless, the symptoms and overall eye health can be considerably enhanced by the incorporation of specific nutrients that are known to benefit the eyes, such as lutein, zeaxanthin, omega-3 fatty acids, and antioxidants.

What Is The Timeframe For The Impact Of Dietary Adjustments On Eye Health?

Eye health can be significantly affected by dietary alterations, which can occur within a few weeks to months. For example, the consumption of leafy greens, such as spinach and kale, which are high in lutein and zeaxanthin, can result in significant enhancements in contrast sensitivity and vision acuity over time. In the same vein, the consistent ingestion of omega-3-rich foods such as salmon or chia seeds can assist in the reduction of inflammation in the eyes and the enhancement of overall eye health within a few months.

Are Supplements Indispensable?

Although a well-balanced diet should ideally provide all the nutrients required for sustaining eye health, supplements can be beneficial, particularly for individuals who may have difficulty obtaining sufficient nutrients from food alone. Nevertheless, it is imperative to seek the advice of a healthcare professional before initiating the use of any supplements, as they have the potential to interact with medications or exacerbate specific health conditions. In addition, supplements should be used in conjunction with a nutritious diet that is abundant in fruits, vegetables, whole cereals, and lean proteins, rather than as a replacement.

Managing Dietary Adjustments In Conjunction With Other Health Conditions

Managing dietary modifications for macular degeneration may necessitate meticulous consideration for individuals with other health conditions, such as diabetes or hypertension.

For instance, individuals with diabetes may require more stringent monitoring of their carbohydrate intake to regulate their blood sugar levels, while those with hypertension may require sodium restriction to preserve adequate blood pressure. It is essential to achieve a balance between managing other health conditions and satisfying the nutritional requirements of macular degeneration to promote overall health.

Managing Sensitivities And Dietary Restrictions

It is imperative to address any dietary restrictions or allergies to guarantee a safe and pleasurable dining experience when implementing a macular degeneration diet. For instance, individuals who are gluten intolerant may need to substitute wheat-based products with gluten-free cereals such as buckwheat or quinoa.

In the same way, individuals with nut allergies can still consume essential nutrients like vitamin E by incorporating alternative sources, such as avocados or sunflower seeds, into their diet. Individuals with macular degeneration can experience a diverse and nutritious diet while avoiding potential allergens by being mindful of dietary restrictions and making appropriate substitutions.

Essential Nutrients For Eye Health

It is essential to consume a diet that is abundant in essential nutrients to maintain good eye health, especially for those who have macular degeneration. These nutrients consist of zinc, selenium, omega-3 fatty acids, lutein, and zeaxanthin, in addition to vitamins A, C, and E. These components are essential for the protection of the eyes from oxidative damage, the preservation of the macula's integrity, and the support of overall eye function.

The roles and sources of vitamins A, C, and E are as follows: They are potent antioxidants that aid in the prevention of oxidative stress in the eyes. Vitamin A promotes the health of the retina and night vision, while vitamin C aids in the production of collagen and safeguards against age-related eye diseases. Vitamin E is essential for the preservation of healthy cells and tissues in the eyes. Carrots, spinach, citrus, almonds, and sunflower seeds are all excellent sources of these vitamins.

Zinc and selenium are indispensable minerals for maintaining eye health. Zinc is essential for the transportation of vitamin A from the liver to the retina, where it is converted into melanin, a protective pigment. Selenium functions as an antioxidant, safeguarding the eyes from the harm from free radicals. Selenium is present in Brazil nuts, fish, eggs, and whole cereals, while foods that are high in zinc include red meat, poultry, seafood, nuts, and legumes.

Omega-3 fatty acids, notably EPA and DHA, which are present in fish oil, are advantageous for eye health. They contribute to the reduction of inflammation and the enhancement of blood flow to the retina, which can delay the progression of macular degeneration. Flaxseeds, chia seeds, and walnuts are plant-based alternatives to omega-3s, which are abundant in fatty fish such as mackerel, sardines, and salmon.

Lutein and zeaxanthin are carotenoids that accumulate in the macula and function as natural filters, shielding the eyes from detrimental blue light and oxidative damage. They are considered super nutrients for the eyes. Additionally, they promote contrast sensitivity and visual acuity. Along with other colorful vegetables such as maize, peppers, and squash, dark leafy greens like kale, spinach, and collard greens are abundant sources of lutein and zeaxanthin.

Incorporating these nutrients into your daily diet can be both effortless and delectable. Begin your day with a spinach and kale smoothie that is rich in lutein and zeaxanthin, as well as vitamins A, C, and E. For lunch, savor a seared salmon salad accompanied by a diverse array of colorful vegetables to enhance antioxidant intake. For a source of zinc and selenium, consume a handful of almonds and seeds as a snack. Additionally, consume roasted vegetables that have been seasoned with olive oil to obtain omega-3 fatty acids. With careful meal preparation, it is effortless to provide your eyes with the necessary nutrients and promote optimal eye health.

CHAPTER FOUR

Foods To Incorporate

The primary components of your diet for macular degeneration should be foods that are high in antioxidants, vitamins, minerals, and omega-3 fatty acids.

Incorporating an abundance of leafy greens, such as spinach, kale, and collard greens, is crucial for ocular health, as they are rich in nutrients such as lutein and zeaxanthin. Additionally, incorporate vibrant fruits and vegetables, including oranges, carrots, berries, and bell peppers, which are abundant in beta-carotene, which is recognized for its ability to promote ocular health, as well as vitamins C and E.

By incorporating fatty fish such as mackerel, sardines, and salmon into your diet, you can obtain a substantial amount of omega-3 fatty acids, which may mitigate the risk of macular degeneration progression. Nuts, seeds, and legumes, including almonds, walnuts, chia seeds, and lentils, are also advantageous due to their elevated levels of antioxidants, vitamins, and minerals.

Finally, choose whole grains such as oats, quinoa, and brown rice to ensure that you are getting the necessary vitamins, minerals, and fiber for optimal health and eye function.

Leafy Greens And Their Advantages

The high concentrations of lutein and zeaxanthin in leafy greens, including spinach, kale, and collard greens, render them indispensable components of a macular degeneration diet. These antioxidants mitigate the risk of macular degeneration progression by safeguarding the eyes from oxidative stress and hazardous light.

By including these greens in your diet, whether in salads, smoothies, or prepared dishes, you guarantee that you are consuming a substantial quantity of these advantageous nutrients. For instance, you may commence your day with a vibrant salad featuring grilled salmon, avocado, and mixed greens, or indulge in a nutrient-rich green smoothie that includes spinach, kale, banana, and almond milk for lunch.

Omega-3 Fatty Acids And Other Omega-3 Sources:

Fatty fish, such as mackerel, sardines, and salmon, are excellent options for incorporating omega-3 fatty acids into your diet. These acids are essential for the preservation of eye health and the reduction of the risk of macular degeneration.

Aim to incorporate a minimum of two servings of fatty fish into your weekly meal plan. If you are not fond of fish, you can also obtain omega-3s from plant-based sources, including walnuts, hemp seeds, chia seeds, and flaxseeds. For instance, you may integrate powdered flaxseeds or chia seeds into homemade granola bars to provide a nutritious and delectable snack or sprinkle them over your morning oatmeal or yogurt.

Colorful Fruits And Vegetables:

Oranges, carrots, berries, and bell peppers are examples of colorful fruits and vegetables that are abundant in beta-carotene, vitamins C and E, and other antioxidants that are crucial for eye health and the prevention of macular degeneration.

To guarantee that you are consuming a diverse array of nutrients, incorporate a variety of colors into your meals. For example, begin your day with a bowl of Greek yogurt and mixed cherries, munch on sliced bell peppers with hummus, and serve roasted carrots and sweet potatoes as a side dish for dinner. In addition to enhancing the flavor and texture of your meals, these vibrant foods also supply essential nutrients that promote eye health.

Legumes, Nuts, and Seeds: Legumes, nuts, and seeds, such as lentils, chia seeds, walnuts, and almonds, are rich in fiber, vitamins, minerals, and antioxidants that can help prevent macular degeneration and promote overall eye health.

By incorporating these nutrient-dense foods into your diet, you can enjoy them as nibbles, add them to salads, soups, or stir-fries, or use them as garnishes for yogurt or oatmeal. For instance, you can incorporate cooked lentils into salads or grain dishes to provide additional protein and fiber or create a trail mix that includes almonds, walnuts, and dried cranberries for a portable and nutritious refreshment.

Foods to Avoid

It is imperative to avoid specific foods that can exacerbate macular degeneration in a macular degeneration diet.

These include foods with a high glycemic index, such as white bread, rice, and sugary treats, which can elevate blood sugar levels and exacerbate ocular inflammation. Furthermore, the consumption of processed meats, including sausage and bacon, can have a detrimental impact on ocular health due to their high levels of sodium and saturated lipids.

Fried foods, such as French fries and fried poultry, should also be avoided due to their high trans fat content, which can cause oxidative stress and retinal injury.

Processed Foods And Their Hazards:

The health of the eyes is often compromised by the presence of unhealthy lipids, sodium, and artificial additives in processed foods. Essential nutrients and fiber are removed from these foods during the extensive processing process, which also introduces hazardous substances.

For example, canned soups and ready-to-eat meals frequently contain elevated sodium levels, which can result in fluid retention and elevated blood pressure, which can have a detrimental effect on ocular health. A higher intake of essential vitamins, minerals, and antioxidants that are beneficial for eye health is guaranteed by choosing whole, unprocessed foods such as fresh fruits, vegetables, and lean proteins.

Eye Health And High-Sugar Foods:

In addition to contributing to systemic health issues such as diabetes, high-sugar foods can also have a detrimental influence on eye health, particularly for individuals with macular degeneration. Blood sugar fluctuations, which can result in inflammation and oxidative stress in the conjunctiva, can be caused by the consumption of foods with a high glycemic index, such as sugary munchies, desserts, and sweetened beverages. This can exacerbate the progression of macular degeneration and elevate the likelihood of vision loss over time.

By selecting whole fruits over processed treats and consuming natural sweeteners such as honey or maple syrup in moderation, it is possible to maintain stable blood sugar levels and promote eye health.

Saturated and trans fats, which are present in foods such as red meat, butter, and processed treats, can contribute to oxidative stress and inflammation in the body, including the eyes. These unhealthy lipids can obstruct arteries and elevate cholesterol levels, thereby obstructing blood flow to the eyes and reducing vision. Replacing saturated lipids with healthier alternatives, such as olive oil, avocado, and fatty fish that are high in omega-3 fatty acids, can aid in the reduction of inflammation and the promotion of overall eye health.

Minimizing trans fat intake and safeguarding against macular degeneration can be achieved by reading food labels and avoiding products that contain hydrogenated or partially hydrogenated oils.

High-Sodium Foods: Consuming high-sodium foods, including processed meats, canned soups, and salty munchies, can result in increased blood pressure and fluid retention, which can have a detrimental effect on ocular health. Overconsumption of sodium can lead to the development of cardiovascular disease and hypertension, which are risk factors for macular degeneration. While enhancing flavor, selecting fresh, homemade dishes that are seasoned with seasonings and spices instead of salt can help reduce sodium intake. Furthermore, the consumption of sodium can be further reduced and ocular health can be promoted by rinsing canned vegetables or selecting low-sodium versions.

CHAPTER FIVE

Breakfast Recipes

Smoothies That Are Rich In Nutrients

Begin your day with a nutritious dose of vitamins and minerals by combining a diverse selection of fruits and vegetables. For instance, a straightforward recipe could consist of a banana, raisins, spinach, and a small amount of almond milk. To guarantee a diverse array of nutrients and identify your preferred flavors, experiment with various combinations.

Breakfast Bowls Made With Whole Grains

Substitute refined grains with whole grains, such as brown rice, quinoa, or oats, to ensure that you have energy for the entire morning. For an additional touch of sweetness, garnish your dish with nuts, seeds, fruits, and a sprinkling of maple syrup or honey.

Additionally, you may incorporate spices such as nutmeg or cinnamon to enhance the flavor.

Healthy Omelets With Leafy Greens

Incorporate leafy greens such as spinach, kale, or Swiss chard to create a nutritious omelet. For an additional burst of flavor and nutrients, incorporate additional vibrant vegetables, including tomatoes, bell peppers, and mushrooms. For preparation, employ avocado oil or olive oil. If preferred, place cheese on top.

Granola With Nuts And Seeds

For a satisfying breakfast or refreshment, prepare your crunchy granola that is packed with almonds and seeds. Combine cereals, almonds, walnuts, pumpkin seeds, sunflower seeds, and a small amount of honey or maple syrup. Spread the mixture evenly onto a baking sheet and bake until it is fragrant and golden brown. For an additional source of protein, pair it with yogurt or milk.

For a nutritious and delightful breakfast parfait, layer Greek yogurt with fresh fruits such as cubed mangoes, sliced bananas, and berries. Add a scattering of crushed almonds or granola between the layers to enhance the texture and crunch. Serve in a transparent glass to emphasize the vibrant layers and relish!

Lunch Recipes For Macular Degeneration Diet

1. Nutrient-Dense Salads with Vibrant Color: Salads are an excellent method for consuming the nutrients that are essential for eye health. Begin with a foundation of dark, verdant greens, such as spinach or kale, and then incorporate colorful vegetables, such as bell peppers, carrots, and tomatoes, to obtain antioxidants such as lutein and zeaxanthin. Add healthful lipids, such as avocado or nuts, to finish it off, which will augment the omega-3 content.

2. Whole Grain Wraps with Lean Protein: Choose whole grain wraps or tortillas that are filled with lean proteins, such as grilled chicken, turkey, or tofu. These are an excellent source of protein that is essential for the preservation of eye health. Include sliced vegetables, leafy greens, and a sprinkling of humus or avocado to enhance the flavor and nutrients.

3. Soups are a nutritious and comforting lunch option. They are also a great source of minerals and vitamins. Select recipes that include a diverse array of colorful vegetables, including spinach, sweet potatoes, and carrots, which are high in vitamins A, C, and E. Incorporate legumes or lentils to obtain plant-based protein and fiber. The flavor and antioxidant content of homemade broth can be improved by infusing it with herbs such as thyme or rosemary.

4. Incorporate a variety of vegetables, including cucumbers, bell peppers, grated carrots, and verdant greens, into whole grain bread or wraps to create vegetable-stuffed sandwiches. These offer an abundance of vitamins and minerals that are essential for eye health. Incorporate condiments such as pesto or humus to enhance the flavor and nutritional value of your dish.

5. Nutritious Grain Bowls: Grain bowls provide an infinite number of opportunities to combine ingredients that are high in nutrients. Begin with a foundation of whole cereals, such as farro, brown rice, or quinoa. Add a variety of colorful vegetables, such as roasted sweet potatoes, broccoli, and cherry tomatoes, and lean proteins like seared salmon, chickpeas, or lean beef, to the top. For an additional burst of flavor and nutritious lipids, drizzle with a homemade vinaigrette or tahini dressing.

Dinner Recipes

Omega-3-Rich Fish Dishes

Try baking salmon with a drizzle of olive oil, a sprinkle of lemon zest, and a fistful of fresh dill for a nutritious and eye-healthy entrée. Serve it alongside a quinoa salad that is seasoned with a mild lemon vinaigrette, diced cucumbers, and cherry tomatoes. This meal is abundant in Omega-3 fatty acids, which are crucial for the promotion of overall eye health and the reduction of inflammation.

Stir-Fries With Vegetables And Leafy Greens

Sauté bell peppers, broccoli, and snap peas with a mixture of kale, spinach, and bok choy to create a fast stir-fry. Season with a dusting of ginger and a dash of soy sauce, and use a tablespoon of sesame oil. Lutein and zeaxanthin, antioxidants that safeguard the eyes from detrimental light exposure, are abundant in this vibrant dish.

Nutrient-Rich Sauces With Whole-Grain Pasta

Prepare a homemade sauce by blending roasted red peppers, tomatoes, garlic, and a small amount of fresh basil. Combine the sauce with cooked whole-grain pasta. For an additional source of nutrients, incorporate sautéed spinach and mushrooms. This meal is a well-balanced source of fiber, vitamins, and minerals that promote overall well-being and eye health.

Stews Of Lean Meat And Vegetables

In a low-sodium chicken bouillon, simmer lean portions of turkey or chicken with a combination of carrots, celery, onions, and butternut squash to create a hearty stew. Incorporate herbs such as rosemary and thyme to enhance the flavor. In addition to being satiating, this stew is also abundant in beta-carotene, a nutrient that is essential for the preservation of excellent vision.

Baking Dishes With Ingredients That Are More Appealing To The Eye

Layer sliced sweet potatoes, zucchini, and tomatoes with a light dusting of mozzarella cheese and fresh herbs such as oregano and basil to create a delectable baked casserole. Bake until the cheese is golden and the vegetables are tender. This dish is abundant in vitamins and antioxidants, which aid in safeguarding the eyes from oxidative stress.

CHAPTER SIX

Seven-Day Meal Plan, Recipes, Ingredients, And Detailed Preparatory Guidelines For Macular Degeneration

The following is a seven-day meal plan for a macular degeneration diet that prioritizes foods that are high in antioxidants, vitamins, and minerals that are specifically designed to promote eye health. Breakfast, lunch, dinner, refreshments, and beverages comprise each day's itinerary.

THE FIRST DAY

Breakfast: Smoothie with Blueberries and Spinach

- **INGREDIENTS:**

o One cup of organic spinach

o 1/2 cup of blueberries

o One banana

o One cup of almond milk

o One tablespoon of chia seeds

• ***PREPARATION:***

1. All ingredients should be combined in a blender.

2. Blend until the mixture is uniform.

3. Serve immediately.

Lunch: Salmon and Avocado Salad

• **INGREDIENTS**:

o One salmon tenderloin

o One minced avocado

o One cup of assorted greens

o 1/2 cucumber, cut

o 1/4 cup cherry tomatoes, halved

o Two tablespoons of olive oil

o One lemon's juice

o Add salt and pepper to taste

• PREPARATION:

1. Grill the salmon fillet until it is fully cooked.

2. Combine the avocado, cherry tomatoes, cucumber, and mixed greens in a sizable basin.

3. Flake the salmon and incorporate it into the salad.

4. Season with salt and pepper, and drizzle with olive oil and lemon juice.

• **INGREDIENTS**:

o Four bell peppers, with the stems removed and the seeds removed

o One cup of quinoa

• 1 1/2 pints of vegetable broth

o One can of black beans, strained and rinsed

o One cup of maize kernels

o 1/2 cup of minced tomatoes

o One teaspoon of cardamom

o One teaspoon of chile powder

o Add salt and pepper to taste

• *PREPARATION:*

1. Turn the oven on to 375°F, or 190°C.

2. Continue to cook the quinoa in a vegetable broth according to the package's instructions.

3. Combine cooked quinoa, black beans, maize, diced tomatoes, cumin, and chile powder in a sizable bowl.

4. Fill the bell peppers with the quinoa mixture.

5. Place the loaded peppers in a baking dish and bake for 25-30 minutes.

Snack: Hummus with carrot sticks

• **INGREDIENTS**:

o Two large carrots, peeled and split into spears

o 1/2 cup of hummus

• *PREPARATION:*

1. Hummus should be served with vegetable spears.

Carrot-orange juice:

• **INGREDIENTS**:

o Four vegetables

o Two peaches

• *PREPARATION:*

1. Combine the carrots and citrus to extract their juice.

2. Mix thoroughly and serve.

THE SECOND DAY

Breakfast: Oatmeal with Nuts and Berries

• **INGREDIENTS**:

o 1/2 cup of dried oats

o One cup of almond milk or water

1/4 cup of assorted berries (strawberries, raspberries, and blueberries)

o One tablespoon of chopped hazelnuts or pecans

o One tablespoon of flaxseeds

• *PREPARATION:*

1. In a saucepan, heat almond milk or water until it reaches a simmer.

2. Add grains and reduce the heat to a simmer. Continue cooking for 5-7 minutes until the mixture thickens.

3. Sprinkle flaxseeds, almonds, and cherries on top.

• **INGREDIENTS**:

o One cup of lentils

o One diced onion

o Two carrots, cut

o Two minced celery stalks

o Three minced garlic cloves

o One can of diced tomatoes

o Four pints of vegetable broth

o One teaspoon of cardamom

o One teaspoon of turmeric

o Add salt and pepper to taste

• PREPARATION:

1. Sauté the onion, carrots, celery, and garlic in a large saucepan until they are tender.

2. Stir in lentils, diced tomatoes, vegetable broth, cumin, and turmeric.

3. Bring the mixture to a boil, then reduce the heat and allow it to simmer for 25-30 minutes.

4. Add salt and pepper to taste.

Dinner: Baked Cod with Sweet Potato Fries

• INGREDIENTS:

o Two cod fillets

o Two sweet potatoes, sliced into slices

o Two tablespoons of olive oil

o One teaspoon of paprika

o One lemon, cut

o Add salt and pepper to taste

• *PREPARATION:*

1. Warm the oven up to 400°F, or 200°C.

2. Combine sweet potato fritters with 1 tablespoon of olive oil, paprika, salt, and pepper. Toss to coat. Distribute the mixture evenly on a baking tray.

3. Bake for 20-25 minutes, rotating once.

4. Arrange the cod fillets on a distinct baking tray. Drizzle with 1 tablespoon of olive oil, season with salt and pepper, and garnish with lemon segments.

5. Bake cod for 12-15 minutes, or until it can be readily flaked with a fork.

• **INGREDIENTS**:

o One apple, cut

o Two tablespoons of almond butter

• *PREPARATION:*

1. Apple segments should be served with almond butter.

Juice: Green Juice

• **INGREDIENTS**:

o One cucumber

o Two stalks of celery

o One green apple

o One fistful of spinach

o One lemon's juice

• *PREPARATION:*

1. Combine all ingredients for juicing.

2. Mix thoroughly and serve.

THIRD DAY

Breakfast: Avocado Toast with Tomato

• **INGREDIENTS**:

o One mature avocado

o One cut tomato

o Two slices of whole-grain bread

o Red pepper flakes, salt, and pepper to flavor

• *PREPARATION:*

1. Toast the bread.

2. The avocado should be mashed and then distributed on the crostini.

3. Add tomato segments to the top.

4. Season with salt, pepper, and red pepper flakes.

Lunch: Spinach and Chickpea Stew

• **INGREDIENTS**:

o One can of legumes, drained and rinsed

o Two cups of fresh spinach

o One diced onion

o Two minced garlic cloves

o One can of diced tomatoes

o Two pints of vegetable broth

o One teaspoon of cardamom

o One teaspoon of paprika

o Add salt and pepper to taste

• *PREPARATION:*

1. Sauté garlic and onion in a sizable saucepan until they are tender.

2. Introduce legumes, spinach, diced tomatoes, vegetable broth, cumin, and paprika.

3. Bring the mixture to a boil, then reduce the heat and allow it to simmer for 15-20 minutes.

4. Add salt and pepper to taste.

Dinner: Broccoli and Quinoa with Grilled Chicken

• INGREDIENTS:

o Two chicken breasts

o One cup of quinoa

o Two cups of broccoli florets

o Two tablespoons of olive oil

o One teaspoon of garlic powder

o Add salt and pepper to taste

• *PREPARATION:*

1. Prepare the quinoa by the instructions provided in the package.

2. Steam broccoli until it is soft.

3. Garlic powder, salt, and pepper are used to season chicken breasts.

4. Grill poultry until it is fully cooked.

5. Serve poultry with broccoli and quinoa.

Snack: A combination of nuts and seeds

• **INGREDIENTS**:

o 1/4 cup of assorted nuts (walnuts, cashews, almonds)

o 1/4 cup of a combination of seeds, including chia, sunflower, and pumpkin

• *PREPARATION:*

1. Combine nuts and seeds and serve.

Apple and beet juice

• **INGREDIENTS**:

o Two beets

o Two peaches

• *PREPARATION:*

1. Combine the juice of pears and vegetables.

2. Mix thoroughly and serve.

THE FOURTH DAY

Breakfast: Greek yogurt with honey and walnuts

• **INGREDIENTS**:

o One cup of Greek yogurt

o One tablespoon of honey

o Two tablespoons of minced walnuts

• *PREPARATION:*

1. Honey and hazelnuts are sprinkled over Greek yogurt.

Lunch: Turkey and Avocado Wrap

• **INGREDIENTS**:

o One whole-grain tortilla

o Three slices of turkey breast

o 1/2 cut avocado

o One cup of assorted greens

o 1/4 cup of shredded carrots

o One tablespoon of hummus

• *PREPARATION:*

1. Apply hummus to the tortilla.

2. Arrange vegetables, avocado, mixed greens, and turkey in a layer.

3. Fold in half and roll up.

Dinner: Brown Rice with Shrimp Stir-Fry

• **INGREDIENTS**:

o One pound of shrimp, skinned and deveined

o Two cups of broccoli florets

o One sliced crimson bell pepper

one carrot, julienned

o Two minced garlic cloves

o Two tablespoons of soy sauce

o One tablespoon of sesame oil

Two tablespoons of brown rice that has been prepared

• PREPARATION:

1. Preheat sesame oil in a sizable skillet over medium-high heat.

2. Add garlic and sauté until it emits a pleasant aroma.

3. Add the shrimp and sauté until they are opaque and pink.

4. Include carrots, bell peppers, and broccoli. Stir-fry the vegetables until they are tender and brown.

5. Incorporate soy sauce.

6. Serve with basmati rice.

Snack: Dark Chocolate with Berries

• **INGREDIENTS**:

o 1/2 cup of a combination of berries, including blueberries, blackberries, and strawberries

o One ounce of dark chocolate

• *PREPARATION:*

1. Dark chocolate should be served with fruit.

Pineapple and kale juice

• **INGREDIENTS**:

o One cup of pineapple segments

o One fistful of kale

o 1/2 cucumber

• PREPARATION:

1. Combine all ingredients for juicing.

2. Mix thoroughly and serve.

DAY FIVE

Breakfast: Mango Chia Seed Pudding

• INGREDIENTS:

o One-quarter cup of chia seeds

• One cup of coconut milk

o One tablespoon of honey

o Diced mango, 1/2

• PREPARATION:

1. Combine honey, coconut milk, and chia seeds in a basin.

2. Place in the refrigerator for a minimum of four hours or overnight.

3. Before serving, garnish with diced mango.

Lunch: Chicken Breast Stuffed with Spinach and Feta

• **INGREDIENTS**:

o Two chicken breasts

o One cup of organic spinach

o Crumbled feta cheese, 1/4 cup

o One tablespoon of olive oil

o Add salt and pepper to taste

• *PREPARATION*:

1. Preheat the oven to 375°F (190°C).

2. Create a cavity in each poultry breast.

3. Fill compartments with feta and vegetables.

4. Use toothpicks to secure.

5. Drizzle with olive oil and season with salt and pepper.

6. Bake the chicken for 25-30 minutes or until it is fully cooked.

Dinner: Vegetable Stir-Fry with Tofu

• **INGREDIENTS**:

o One cubed slab of firm tofu

o One cup of snap peas

o One sliced crimson bell pepper

one carrot, julienned

o Two minced garlic cloves

o Two tablespoons of soy sauce

o One tablespoon of sesame oil

Two tablespoons of brown rice that has been prepared

• *PREPARATION:*

1. In a sizable skillet, heat sesame oil over medium-high heat.

2. Add garlic and sauté until it emits a pleasant aroma.

3. Add the tofu and continue cooking until it turns a golden brown color.

4. Include carrots, bell peppers, and snap peas. Stir-fry the vegetables until they are tender and brown.

5. Incorporate soy sauce.

6. Serve with basmati rice.

- **INGREDIENTS**:

o Three celery stalks, sliced into pieces

o Two tablespoons of peanut butter

- *PREPARATION:*

1. Peanut butter should be served with celery stalks.

Apple and spinach juice

- **INGREDIENTS**:

o Two peaches

o One fistful of spinach

- *PREPARATION:*

1. Combine the juice of pears and spinach.

2. Mix thoroughly and serve.

SIXTH DAY

• **INGREDIENTS**:

o One cup of whole-grain flour

o One tablespoon of baking powder

o One tablespoon of sugar

o 1/2 teaspoon of salt

o One cup of almond milk

o One egg

o Two tablespoons of olive oil

o 1/2 cup of blueberries

• PREPARATION:

1. Combine flour, baking powder, sugar, and salt in a basin.

2. Whisk almond milk, egg, and olive oil in a separate basin.

3. Mix the dry ingredients with the liquid ingredients until they are fully incorporated.

4. Incorporate blueberries by folding.

5. Place a non-stick skillet over medium heat and pour 1/4 cup of batter into it for each pancake.

6. Cook until bubbles appear on the surface, then rotate and continue cooking until the surface is golden brown.

Mediterranean Quinoa Salad for Lunch

• INGREDIENTS:

o One cup of prepared quinoa

o. Half a cup of cherry tomatoes

o Diced cucumber, 1/4 cup

o One-quarter cup of diced kalamata olives

1/4 cup of finely sliced red onion

o Crumbled feta cheese, 1/4 cup

o Two tablespoons of olive oil

o One lemon's juice

o Add salt and pepper to taste

• *PREPARATION:*

1. Combine quinoa, cucumber, olives, red onion, cherry tomatoes, and feta cheese in a sizable basin.

2. Season with salt and pepper, and drizzle with olive oil and lemon juice.

3. Combine by tossing.

• **INGREDIENTS**:

o Two fillets of tilapia

o One bundle of asparagus, trimmed

o Two tablespoons of olive oil

o One lemon, cut

o Add salt and pepper to taste

• *PREPARATION:*

1. Set oven temperature to 400°F, or 200°C.

2. Arrange asparagus and tilapia fillets on a baking tray.

3. Season with salt and pepper and drizzle with olive oil.

4. Add lemon segments to the top.

5. Bake for 12-15 minutes, or until the salmon can be readily flaked with a fork.

• **INGREDIENTS**:

o One sliced crimson bell pepper

o 1/2 cup of avocado

• *PREPARATION:*

1. Guacamole should be served alongside bell pepper segments.

Carrot, apple, and ginger juice

• **INGREDIENTS**:

o Three vegetables

o Two peaches

o One-inch slice of ginger

• PREPARATION:

1. Combine carrots, pears, and ginger in a juicer.

2. Mix thoroughly and serve.

SEVENTH DAY

Breakfast: Smoothie Bowl

• INGREDIENTS:

o One banana

o 1/2 cup of chilled fruit

o 1/2 cup of Greek yogurt

o 1/2 cup of almond milk

o One tablespoon of chia seeds

o One tablespoon of granola

• *PREPARATION:*

1. Blend almond milk, frozen berries, Greek yogurt, and a banana in a blender.

2. Blend until the mixture is uniform.

3. Transfer the mixture to a vessel and garnish with granola and chia seeds.

Lunch: Veggie Wrap

• **INGREDIENTS**:

o One whole-grain tortilla

o 1/2 cup of hummus

o 1/4 cup of shredded carrots

1/4 cup of diced cucumber

o 1/4 cup of bell pepper segments

o 1/4 cup of spinach fronds

• PREPARATION:

1. Apply hummus to the tortilla.

2. Arrange carrots, cucumber, bell pepper, and spinach in a layer.

3. Fold in half and roll up.

Dinner: Black Bean and Grilled Vegetable Tacos

• INGREDIENTS:

o One zucchini, cut

o One sliced crimson bell pepper

o One sliced red onion

o One can of black beans, strained and rinsed

o One tablespoon of olive oil

o One teaspoon of cardamom

o One teaspoon of chile powder

o Eight mini maize tortillas

o One-quarter cup of minced cilantro

o 1/2 cup of salsa

• *PREPARATION:*

1. Preheat the grill to medium-high fire.

2. Combine zucchini, bell pepper, and onion with chile powder, cumin, and olive oil.

3. Grill vegetables until they are barely charred and tender.

4. Tortillas that are still warm from the griddle.

5. Fill tortillas with black beans and grilled vegetables.

6. Sprinkle minced cilantro and salsa on top.

- **INGREDIENTS**:

o One split pear

o 1/4 cup of ricotta cheese

- *PREPARATION:*

1. Ricotta cheese should be served alongside pear segments.

Spinach and pineapple juice

- **INGREDIENTS**:

o One fistful of spinach

o One cup of pineapple segments

o 1/2 cucumber

• PREPARATION:

1. Combine cucumber, pineapple, and spinach in a juicer.

2. Mix thoroughly and serve.

A diverse selection of nutrient-dense foods is incorporated into this dietary plan to promote eye health and overall well-being. Have fun!

<u>CHAPTER SEVEN</u>

7 Procedural Dessert Recipes For The Macular Degeneration Diet And Guidelines

Age-related macular degeneration (AMD) is a prevalent eye condition that can result in vision loss in elderly individuals. AMD can be effectively managed by adhering to a diet that is abundant in antioxidants, vitamins, and minerals. Incorporating these nutrients into desserts can be a delightful experience. The following are seven dessert recipes that are specifically designed for a macular degeneration diet, as well as some important guidelines to keep in mind.

Dietary Recommendations For Macular Degeneration

1. Concentrate on Antioxidants: Consuming foods that are rich in zinc, beta-carotene, and vitamins C

and E can mitigate the risk of AMD. Nuts, seeds, fruits, and vegetables comprise this category.

2. Include Omega-3 Fatty Acids: Omega-3s, which are present in flaxseeds and fish, are crucial for eye health.

3. Restrict the Consumption of Saturated Fats and Sugars: A high intake of saturated fats and sugars can exacerbate AMD. Select natural sweeteners and healthful lipids.

4. Choose whole grains: In comparison to refined grains, whole grains contain a greater amount of fiber and nutrients.

1. BLUEBERRY CHIA SEED PUDDING

INGREDIENTS:

• One cup of almond milk

• 1/4 cup of chia seeds

• One cup of organic blueberries

• 1-2 teaspoons of maple syrup or honey

• 1/2 teaspoon of vanilla extract

STEPS:

1. Combine almond milk, chia seeds, honey, and vanilla extract in a basin.

2. Stir the mixture thoroughly and place it in the refrigerator for a minimum of four hours or overnight.

3. Blend fresh blueberries into a sauce before serving.

4. Layer the blueberry sauce over the chia pudding in serving glasses.

5. Add a few whole blueberries as a garnish.

Nutritional Highlight: Blueberries are abundant in antioxidants, particularly vitamin C and vitamin E, which are advantageous for eye health.

2. CHOCOLATE AVOCADO MOUSSE

INGREDIENTS:

• Two mature avocados

• 1/4 cup of cocoa powder

• 1/4 cup of maple syrup or honey

• One teaspoon of vanilla extract

• A mere sprinkle of salt

STEPS:

1. Transfer the avocado interior to a blender.

2. Honey, cocoa powder, vanilla extract, and salt should be incorporated.

3. Blend until the mixture is velvety and smooth.

4. Before serving, allow the dish to cool in the refrigerator for one hour.

Nutritional Highlight: Avocados are an excellent source of lutein and zeaxanthin, which are antioxidants that are essential for eye health.

3. BERRY QUINOA PARFAIT

INGREDIENTS:

• One cup of prepared quinoa

• One cup of Greek yogurt

• One cup of a combination of berries, including raspberries, blueberries, and strawberries

• 1-2 teaspoons of agave nectar or honey

• 1/2 teaspoon of cinnamon

STEPS:

1. Combine the cooked quinoa with cinnamon and honey.

2. Layer the quinoa, Greek yogurt, and assorted berries in a glass.

3. Repeat the layers and garnish with a few berries.

Nutritional Highlight: Quinoa is a source of protein and fiber, while berries are an abundant source of antioxidants.

4. BROWNIES MADE WITH SWEET POTATOES

INGREDIENTS:

• One cup of mashed sweet potatoes

• 1/2 cup of almond butter

• 1/4 cup of cocoa powder

• 1/4 cup of maple syrup or honey

• One teaspoon of vanilla extract

• 1/2 teaspoon of baking soda

STEPS:

1. Set the oven's temperature to 175°C/350°F.

2. Combine all ingredients in a basin until they are thoroughly mixed.

3. Transfer the batter to a baking pan that has been greased.

4. Bake for 20-25 minutes or until a toothpick inserted into the center of the cake emerges clean.

5. Let cool completely before cutting into squares.

Nutritional Highlight: Beta-carotene, which is essential for ocular health, is abundant in sweet potatoes and is converted to vitamin A in the body.

INGREDIENTS:

• Two mature mangoes, trimmed and cubed

• 1/2 cup of coconut milk

• Two tablespoons of maple syrup or honey

• The juice of one citrus

STEPS:

1. All ingredients should be blended until they are homogeneous.

2. Transfer the mixture to a container that is suitable for freezing.

3. Stir occasionally while freezing for a minimum of four hours.

4. Chill and serve.

Nutritional Highlight: Mangoes are abundant in vitamin A and vitamin C, both of which are crucial for eye health.

6. SMOOTHIE MADE WITH SPINACH AND BANANAS

INGREDIENTS:

• One mature banana

• One cup of fresh spinach leaves

• One-half cup of Greek yogurt

• One-half cup of almond milk

• One tablespoon of flaxseeds

• One teaspoon of honey (optional)

STEPS:

1. All ingredients should be combined in a blender.

2. Blend until the mixture is uniform.

3. Pour the mixture into glasses and serve immediately.

Nutritional Highlight: Spinach is an excellent source of zeaxanthin and lutein, which are essential for safeguarding the eyes from hazardous radiation.

7. SALAD WITH APPLES AND WALNUTS

INGREDIENTS:

• Two apples, cored and diced

• Chopped walnuts, 1/2 cup

• 1/4 cup of raisins

• One tablespoon of agave nectar or honey

• One teaspoon of cinnamon

• The juice of one lemon

STEPS:

1. To prevent discoloration, combine the diced apples with lemon juice in a basin.

2. Stir in honey, hazelnuts, raisins, and cinnamon.

3. Mix thoroughly and refrigerate for 30 minutes before serving.

Apples and walnuts are rich in antioxidants, and walnuts also contain omega-3 fatty acids.

In summary, the incorporation of nutrient-dense delicacies into one's diet can be a delectable method of promoting eye health and managing macular degeneration. These recipes emphasize the importance of antioxidants, vitamins, and minerals in the preservation of good vision while prohibiting the consumption of excessive carbohydrates and unhealthy lipids. For optimal eye health, incorporate these delights into a well-balanced diet. Please enjoy.

CHAPTER EIGHT

Seven Smoothies Procedural Recipes For Macular Degeneration And Guidelines

Diet can have an impact on macular degeneration, a primary cause of vision loss. Supporting eye health can be achieved by incorporating nutrient-rich smoothies into your daily routine. Seven smoothie recipes have been developed with macular degeneration in mind, each of which is abundant in antioxidants, vitamins, and minerals that enhance eye health.

Smoothie Preparation Guidelines

1. Ingredient Selection: To optimize nutrient intake, prioritize the use of fresh, organic ingredients whenever feasible. Concentrate on seeds that are abundant in omega-3 fatty acids, colorful fruits, and dark verdant greens.

2. Balance: Each smoothie must contain an appropriate proportion of fruits and vegetables. Aim for a 3:1 ratio of fruits to vegetables.

3. Liquid Base: To prevent the addition of superfluous carbohydrates and to enhance the nutritional value, utilize unsweetened almond milk, coconut water, or green tea as a base.

4. Sweeteners: If additional sweetness is required, consider natural sources such as stevia, dates, or honey.

5. Preparation: The ingredients should be blended until they are homogeneous. To achieve the desired consistency, it may be necessary to modify the liquid quantity when utilizing frozen fruits or vegetables.

6. Serving: Consume immediately to guarantee optimal nutrient assimilation.

INGREDIENTS:

• One cup of organic kale

• One cup of blueberries

• One banana

• One tablespoon of chia seeds

• One cup of strained almond milk

• One teaspoon of honey (optional)

STEPS:

1. Thoroughly rinse the blueberries and kale.

2. Combine the kale, blueberries, banana, and chia seeds in the blender.

3. Pour the almond milk into the container.

4. Blend until the mixture is uniform. Add honey if desired and blend once more.

5. Serve immediately.

2. MANGO AND SPINACH MAGIC

INGREDIENTS:

• One cup of fresh spinach

• One cup of chilled mango segments

• One orange, skinned and segmented

• One tablespoon of flax seeds

• One cup of coconut water

STEPS:

1. Thoroughly rinse the broccoli.

2. Incorporate spinach, mango chunks, orange segments, and flax seeds into the blender.

3. Pour the coconut water into the container.

4. Blend until the mixture is uniform.

5. Serve immediately.

3. AVOCADO AND BERRY SUPPLEMENT

INGREDIENTS:

• One-half of a mature avocado

• One-half cup of strawberries

• 1/2 cup of raspberries

• One tablespoon of hemp seeds

• One cup of chilled green tea

STEPS:

1. Place the avocado flesh in the blender by scooping it out.

2. Incorporate hemp seeds, raspberries, and strawberries.

3. Add the cooled green tea.

4. Blend until the mixture is uniform.

5. Serve immediately.

4. CARROT AND ORANGE ZEST

INGREDIENTS:

• 1 cup grated carrots

• One orange, skinned and segmented

• One-half of a banana

• 1 teaspoonful pumpkin seeds

• One cup of strained almond milk

1. If not already done, grate the carrots.

2. Incorporate carrots, orange segments, bananas, and pumpkin seeds into the blender.

3. Pour the almond milk into the container.

4. Blend until the mixture is uniform.

5. Serve immediately.

5. APPLE AND SWEET POTATO FUSION

INGREDIENTS:

• One-half cup of sweet potato that has been cooked

• One apple, cored and sliced

• 1/2 teaspoon of cinnamon

• One tablespoon of sunflower seeds

• One cup of strained almond milk

STEPS:

1. Cook and allow the sweet potato to cool.

2. Combine the sweet potato, apple, cinnamon, and sunflower seeds in the blender.

3. Pour the almond milk into the container.

4. Blend until the mixture is uniform.

5. Serve immediately.

6. BEET AND BERRY BLAST

INGREDIENTS:

• One small beet, peeled and chopped

• One-half cup of blueberries

• One-half cup of strawberries

• One tablespoon of chia seeds

• One cup of coconut Water

STEPS:

1. Prepare the beet by peeling and chopping it.

2. Add blueberries, strawberries, beets, and chia seeds to the blender.

3. Pour the coconut water into the container.

4. Blend until the mixture is uniform.

5. Serve immediately.

7. GREEN APPLE AND KIWI PUNCH

INGREDIENTS:

• One green apple, cored and sliced

• Two kiwis, peeled and chopped

• One cup of fresh spinach

• One tablespoon of flax seeds

• One cup of strained almond milk

STEPS:

1. Chop and core the apple.

2. Peel and chop the kiwis.

3. Add apple, kiwis, spinach, and flax seeds to the blender.

4. Pour the almond milk into the container.

5. Blend until the mixture is uniform.

6. Serve immediately.

Nutritional Highlights

• Leafy Greens: Contain lutein and zeaxanthin, which are antioxidants that are crucial for eye health.

• Berries: They are rich in vitamins C and E, which shield the body from oxidative stress.

• Seeds: Omega-3 fatty acids are present in chia, flax, and hemp seeds, which can mitigate inflammation.

• Orange and Yellow Vegetables: Beta-carotene, which is essential for vision, is abundant in carrots and sweet potatoes.

• Green tea is a source of antioxidants that promote the overall health of the eye.

By incorporating these smoothies into your diet, you can experience delectable, nutrient-rich beverages and support your eye health.

CHAPTER NINE

Quantity Desserts And Snacks

If you are seeking a nutritious and satisfying indulgence, prioritize foods that are low in added sugars and high in antioxidants to promote eye health. For a sweeter taste, incorporate dried cranberries and dark chocolate chunks into a trail mix that includes almonds, walnuts, and pumpkin seeds. Natural sugars and fiber are provided by fruit-based delicacies, such as baked pears with a sprinkling of cinnamon. Smoothie dishes containing frozen berries, spinach, and a small amount of almond milk may be garnished with sliced kiwi and chia seeds.

For a low-sugar delicacy, consider baking oatmeal biscuits that are sweetened with mashed bananas and a small amount of dark chocolate morsels.

Combine nuts and seeds with colorful fruits and vegetables to create antioxidant-rich treats. Cut bell peppers, carrots, and cucumbers into thin slices for dipping in hummus, which is abundant in vitamins and minerals.

A small serving of blueberries, which are rich in antioxidants, when combined with a sprinkling of almonds, provides a combination of sweet and savory flavors. A fast guacamole can be prepared with avocados and lime juice, and it can be served with whole grain crackers. For a fast, nutritious snack, maintain a supply of easily accessible alternatives, such as dried apricots and a small amount of dark chocolate.

Nut And Seed Blends

Formulate a nutritious nut and seed mixture that is ideal for on-the-go nibbling. For a hint of sweetness, combine a half-cup of desiccated goji berries or raisins with a cup each of raw almonds, cashews, and sunflower seeds.

Add a small amount of chia seeds and pumpkin seeds, which are both rich in omega-3 fatty acids. This mixture can be transported to work in a container or consumed as a rapid, energy-boosting refreshment.

To enhance the flavor, you may also delicately season it with a sprinkle of sea salt or a dash of cinnamon.

Desserts That Are Based On Fruit

Transform fresh fruits into delectable and nutritious delicacies that satiate your sweet tooth without the addition of sugar. Consider preparing a fruit salad that includes a diverse selection of berries, melons, and kiwi. To enhance its freshness, drench it with honey and garnish it with mint leaves.

A warm and comforting delicacy is achieved by baking pears with a sprinkling of cinnamon and a dollop of Greek yogurt. An additional alternative is to freeze banana segments and puree them until they are smooth, resulting in a dairy-free, creamy ice cream substitute.

For an additional indulgence, sprinkle a few shavings of dark chocolate on top.

Smoothie Bowls

Smoothie dishes are a nutrient-rich and adaptable choice for breakfast or dessert. Combine a banana, a fistful of frozen strawberries, a cup of spinach, and a small amount of almond milk in a blender until the mixture is homogeneous. Pour the mixture into a bowl and garnish with granola, chia seeds, and fresh berries to enhance the texture and provide additional nutrients.

For a tropical variation, combine coconut milk with frozen mango and pineapple, and then garnish with shredded coconut and kiwi segments.

Smoothie bowls can be effortlessly personalized to incorporate your preferred fruits and garnishes, resulting in a visually appealing and delectable dish.

Low-Sugar Baked Goods

Utilize natural sweeteners and nutrient-dense ingredients to prepare nutritious delights that are low in sugar but high in flavor. Prepare a quantity of banana oatmeal muffins by mashing mature bananas and combining them with oats, a small amount of honey, and a fistful of walnuts.

For a chocolate dose, bake brownies with almond flour and sweeten with dates or a small amount of maple syrup. For a low-sugar, comforting nibble, apple cinnamon muffins can be made with whole wheat flour and unsweetened applesauce. These delights are ideal for satisfying appetites while simultaneously promoting eye health.

Conclusion

A diet that is specifically designed for macular degeneration (MD) is essential for the management and potential halting of the progression of this eye condition. The significance of particular nutrients that promote eye health is emphasized in the conclusion of the macular degeneration diet.

Leafy greens, citrus fruits, almonds, and seeds are all sources of key components, including antioxidants like zinc, beta-carotene, and vitamins C and E. Omega-3 fatty acids, which are found in oily fish such as mackerel and salmon, are also essential for the maintenance of retinal health and the reduction of inflammation.

A sufficient intake of carotenoids, such as lutein and zeaxanthin, is guaranteed by incorporating a diverse selection of vibrant fruits and vegetables. These compounds are recognized for their ability to safeguard the macula by filtering hazardous blue light.

Furthermore, it is advised to consume a diet that is well-balanced and low in cholesterol and saturated fats to enhance overall vascular health, which in turn enhances ocular circulation.

Although macular degeneration cannot be cured by diet alone, it is a substantial complementary treatment to other methods.

The efficacy of dietary interventions is further enhanced by the prevention of smoking, the maintenance of a healthy weight, and the management of underlying health conditions, such as hypertension and diabetes. Individuals with MD may enhance their quality of life and vision by adhering to these dietary recommendations.

THE END